PLANT-BASED OSTEOPOROSIS DIET COOKBOOK

"The Ultimate Guide with High-Protein Recipes and Exercises to Naturally Prevent and Reverse Bone Loss"

Dayna G. Murphy

Copyright © 2024 by Dayna G. Murphy

All rights reserved.

Disclaimer: The information provided in this book is for educational purposes only and is not intended as a substitute for professional medical advice, diagnosis, or treatment.

GAIN ACCESS TO OTHER BOOKS BY ME

TABLE OF CONTENTS

INTRODUCTION

Welcome to Nourish Your Bones

Purpose of the Book:

The **"Plant-Based Osteoporosis Diet Cookbook"** is designed to empower individuals with a comprehensive guide to adopting a plant-based lifestyle that supports optimal bone health. The key purposes of this book include:

1. Educating About Osteoporosis:

- Provide clear and accessible information about osteoporosis, its causes, and the significance of nutrition in maintaining strong and healthy bones.

2. Promoting Plant-Based Nutrition:

- Showcase the benefits of a plant-based diet in preventing and managing osteoporosis, emphasizing nutrient-rich foods that contribute to bone health.

3. Offering Practical Guidance:

- Provide practical tips on incorporating essential nutrients like calcium, vitamin D, and magnesium into everyday meals to ensure a well-balanced and bone-friendly diet.

4. Highlighting Scientific Evidence:

- Present scientific evidence supporting the effectiveness of plant-based diets in promoting bone health, backed by research and studies.

5. Encouraging a Holistic Lifestyle:

- Emphasize the role of physical activity, mindfulness, and stress management in maintaining overall well-being, complementing the dietary recommendations.

How to Use This Cookbook:

1. Educational Sections:

- Begin by reading the introductory sections on osteoporosis, causes, and risk factors. Familiarize yourself with the importance of nutrition for bone health.

2. Nutrient Charts:

- Refer to the nutrient charts for quick information on calcium-rich, vitamin D-rich, and magnesium-rich foods. Use these charts as a reference when planning your meals.

3. Meal Plans:

- Explore the sample meal plans provided for inspiration. These plans offer a variety of plant-based recipes rich in bone-essential nutrients. Adjust portion sizes based on individual needs.

4. Recipes:

- Dive into the cookbook's recipe section, where you'll find a collection of delicious plant-based dishes designed specifically for promoting bone health. Each recipe includes detailed instructions and nutrient information.

5. Essential Ingredients and Tools:

- Familiarize yourself with the essential ingredients and kitchen tools recommended for preparing the recipes in this cookbook. This section ensures you have everything you need to get started.

6. Breakfast Boosters, Lunch Ideas, Dinner Delights, Snacks, and Desserts:

- Explore these dedicated sections for a diverse range of recipes tailored to different times of the day. From energizing breakfasts to satisfying dinners and delightful desserts, this cookbook has you covered.

7. Incorporating Calcium-Rich Foods:

- Follow the practical tips on incorporating calcium-rich foods into your diet for optimal absorption. Learn about nutrient interactions and find a balance that works for you.

8. Physical Activity and Mindfulness:

- Understand the connection between physical activity, mindfulness, and bone health. Learn how these lifestyle factors contribute to overall well-being.

9. Celebrating Your Journey:

- Wrap up your exploration of the cookbook by celebrating your achievements. Reflect on your progress, set new goals, and continue your plant-based journey towards healthier bones.

This cookbook is a tool to guide and inspire you on your path to better bone health through a plant-based lifestyle. Feel free to customize the recipes, adjust the meal plans, and make this cookbook your own as you embark on this exciting and healthful journey.

CHAPTER 1: UNDERSTANDING OSTEOPOROSIS

Introduction to Osteoporosis

What is Osteoporosis?

Osteoporosis is a medical condition characterized by the weakening of bones, making them fragile and more susceptible to fractures. This occurs when the density and quality of bone are reduced. Bones naturally undergo a continuous process of formation and resorption, but in individuals with osteoporosis, the creation of new bone doesn't keep up with the removal of old bone.

Causes and Risk Factors

1. Aging:

- Osteoporosis is more common in older adults as bone density tends to decrease with age.

2. Hormonal Changes:

- Postmenopausal women are at a higher risk due to a decrease in estrogen levels, which plays a protective role in bone health.

3. Family History:

- A family history of osteoporosis increases the likelihood of developing the condition.

4. Low Body Weight:

- Individuals with a low body mass index (BMI) may have less bone mass and are at a higher risk.

5. Certain Medications:

- Long-term use of corticosteroids, thyroid medications, and some anticonvulsants can contribute to bone loss.

6. Dietary Factors:

- Inadequate intake of calcium and vitamin D, essential for bone health, can increase the risk of osteoporosis.

7. Sedentary Lifestyle:

- Lack of weight-bearing exercises and physical activity can lead to bone loss.

8. Medical Conditions:

- Certain medical conditions, such as rheumatoid arthritis, gastrointestinal disorders, and hormonal disorders, can increase the risk of osteoporosis.

Importance of Nutrition for Bone Health

1. Calcium:

- Calcium is a crucial mineral for bone health. It's essential for the formation and maintenance of strong bones.

2. Vitamin D:

- Vitamin D is necessary for the absorption of calcium in the intestines. Sunlight exposure is a natural source of vitamin D, and it is also found in some foods.

3. Protein:

- Protein is important for bone formation, and a deficiency can impair the body's ability to build and repair bones.

4. Phosphorus:

- Phosphorus, along with calcium, contributes to bone strength. Maintaining a balance between these two minerals is crucial.

5. Magnesium:

- Magnesium is involved in bone mineralization and helps regulate calcium levels.

6. Vitamin K:

- Vitamin K plays a role in bone metabolism and helps in the synthesis of proteins involved in bone mineralization.

7. Omega-3 Fatty Acids:

- Found in certain plant-based sources, omega-3 fatty acids may have anti-inflammatory effects that support bone health.

A balanced and nutrient-rich diet, combined with a healthy lifestyle, can significantly contribute to maintaining strong and healthy bones, reducing the risk of osteoporosis. Regular exercise, especially weight-bearing activities, is also crucial for bone density and overall bone health.

The Role of Plant-Based Diets

Benefits of Plant-Based Eating:

1. Heart Health:

- Plant-based diets are associated with lower levels of saturated fats and cholesterol, contributing to a reduced risk of heart disease. High fiber content in plant foods also supports heart health.

2. Weight Management:

- Plant-based diets tend to be lower in calorie density and fat, making them effective for weight management and weight loss. The emphasis on whole, nutrient-dense foods helps control calorie intake.

3. Diabetes Management:

- Plant-based diets have been linked to improved insulin sensitivity and better blood sugar control, reducing the risk of type 2 diabetes and supporting diabetes management.

4. Cancer Prevention:

- Antioxidants and phytochemicals found in plant-based foods have been associated with a lower risk of certain cancers. The fiber content may also contribute to a reduced risk of colorectal cancer.

5. Improved Digestive Health:

- The high fiber content in plant foods promotes a healthy digestive system by preventing constipation and supporting the growth of beneficial gut bacteria.

6. Reduced Inflammation:

- Plant-based diets, rich in anti-inflammatory compounds, may help reduce inflammation in the body, lowering the risk of chronic inflammatory conditions.

7. Lower Blood Pressure:

- The potassium-rich nature of many plant foods, along with reduced sodium intake, supports lower blood pressure, reducing the risk of hypertension and cardiovascular diseases.

8. Longevity:

- Some studies suggest that plant-based diets are associated with increased life expectancy and a reduced risk of premature mortality.

Key Nutrients for Bone Health:

1. Calcium:

- Essential for bone mineralization, calcium is abundant in plant sources such as leafy green vegetables (kale, bok choy), fortified plant-based milk, and tofu.

2. Vitamin D:

- Critical for calcium absorption, vitamin D can be obtained through sun exposure and fortified plant-based sources like fortified cereals and plant-based milk.

3. Magnesium:

- Plays a crucial role in bone structure and function. Plant-based sources of magnesium include nuts, seeds, whole grains, and leafy green vegetables.

4. Vitamin K:

- Necessary for bone metabolism, vitamin K is found in abundance in leafy green vegetables, broccoli, Brussels sprouts, and other green veggies.

5. Protein:

- Important for bone formation, plant-based protein sources include legumes (beans, lentils), tofu, tempeh, quinoa, and nuts.

6. Omega-3 Fatty Acids:

- Found in chia seeds, flaxseeds, hemp seeds, and walnuts, omega-3 fatty acids may contribute to bone health through their anti-inflammatory effects.

Scientific Evidence Supporting Plant-Based Diets:

1. Bone Health Studies:

- Research indicates that a well-planned plant-based diet can provide sufficient nutrients for bone health, and some studies suggest a positive association between plant-based diets and bone mineral density.

2. Cardiovascular Health:

- Numerous studies support the cardiovascular benefits of plant-based diets, including lower cholesterol levels, reduced blood pressure, and a decreased risk of heart disease.

3. Cancer Prevention Research:

- Observational studies have shown that plant-based diets rich in fruits, vegetables, and whole grains may contribute to a lower risk of certain cancers.

4. Diabetes Management:

- Plant-based diets, particularly those emphasizing whole, unprocessed foods, have been linked to a reduced risk of type 2 diabetes and improved glycemic control in individuals with diabetes.

5. Inflammatory Conditions:

- Some research suggests that plant-based diets may help mitigate chronic inflammatory conditions due to their anti-inflammatory properties.

6. Longevity Studies:

- Several studies suggest that adopting plant-based diets may be associated with increased life expectancy and a lower risk of chronic diseases, contributing to overall longevity.

CHAPTER 2: GETTING STARTED WITH A PLANT-BASED LIFESTYLE

Transitioning to a Plant-Based Diet

Gradual Changes and Adjustments:

1. Start Small:

- Begin by making small changes to your diet and lifestyle. This could involve incorporating one plant-based meal per day or increasing your daily water intake.

2. Incremental Adjustments:

- Gradually increase the proportion of plant-based foods in your meals. For example, try replacing meat with plant-based proteins in a few meals each week.

3. Experiment with Recipes:

- Explore new plant-based recipes and find ones that you enjoy. Experimenting with flavors and textures can make the transition more enjoyable.

4. Meal Planning:

- Plan your meals for the week, incorporating a variety of plant-based foods. This can help you make intentional choices and reduce reliance on processed or convenience foods.

5. Educate Yourself:

- Learn about the nutritional benefits of different plant-based foods. Understanding the positive impact on your health can motivate you to make gradual changes.

1. Lack of Protein:

- **Misconception:** A common belief is that plant-based diets lack sufficient protein.
- **Clarification:** Plant-based sources like beans, lentils, tofu, and quinoa provide ample protein. A well-balanced plant-based diet can meet protein needs.

2. Inadequate Nutrients:

- **Misconception:** Concerns about missing essential nutrients like calcium and vitamin B12.

- **Clarification:** Plant-based sources, fortified foods, and supplements can address nutrient needs. Proper planning ensures a well-rounded diet.

3. Bland and Boring Meals:

- **Misconception:** Some may think that plant-based meals are bland and unappealing.
- **Clarification:** Plant-based cooking can be diverse and flavorful. Explore herbs, spices, and cooking techniques to enhance taste.

4. Difficulty in Social Situations:

- **Misconception:** Difficulty in social gatherings due to limited plant-based options.
- **Clarification:** Many restaurants offer plant-based choices, and you can communicate your dietary preferences ahead of time. Bring plant-based dishes to share at gatherings.

Overcoming Challenges:

1. Support System:

- Seek support from friends, family, or online communities. Share your journey and exchange tips with others who have embraced a plant-based lifestyle.

2. Educate Others:

- Educate those around you about the benefits of a plant-based diet. This can dispel misconceptions and garner support from those close to you.

3. Meal Prep:

- Plan and prepare plant-based meals in advance. Having nutritious options readily available can prevent resorting to less healthy choices.

4. Flexibility:

- Be flexible and open to trying new foods and recipes. Embrace the variety that a plant-based diet offers, and don't be afraid to experiment.

5. Gradual Transition:

- If transitioning from a non-plant-based diet, consider a gradual approach. Allow time for your taste buds and digestive system to adjust to new foods.

6. Focus on Whole Foods:

- Prioritize whole, minimally processed foods. This ensures a nutrient-dense diet and minimizes reliance on heavily processed plant-based alternatives.

7. Professional Guidance:

- Consult with a registered dietitian or nutritionist for personalized guidance. They can help address concerns, provide meal plans, and ensure nutritional adequacy.

Remember, adopting a plant-based lifestyle is a personal journey. Be patient with yourself, celebrate your successes, and continuously reassess and adjust as needed. Every small change contributes to a healthier, more sustainable lifestyle.

Building a Plant-Based Pantry

Essential Ingredients:

1. Leafy Greens:

- Kale, spinach, collard greens, and Swiss chard provide essential vitamins and minerals like calcium and vitamin K.

2. Tofu and Tempeh:

- Rich sources of plant-based protein and calcium, versatile for various recipes.

3. Beans and Lentils:

- High in protein, fiber, and minerals like iron and magnesium, contributing to a well-rounded plant-based diet.

4. Whole Grains:

- Quinoa, brown rice, oats, and whole wheat provide complex carbohydrates, fiber, and essential nutrients.

5. Nuts and Seeds:

- Almonds, walnuts, chia seeds, flaxseeds, and sunflower seeds offer healthy fats, protein, and minerals like calcium and magnesium.

6. Fortified Plant-Based Milk:

- Almond, soy, or oat milk fortified with calcium and vitamin D for essential bone health.

7. Colorful Vegetables:

- Bell peppers, tomatoes, carrots, broccoli, and other colorful veggies provide a range of vitamins, antioxidants, and fiber.

8. Herbs and Spices:

- Fresh herbs like basil, cilantro, and parsley, along with spices such as turmeric, cumin, and garlic, add flavor and nutritional benefits.

9. Whole Fruits:

- Apples, berries, citrus fruits, and bananas offer natural sweetness, vitamins, and antioxidants.

10. Whole-Grain Pasta and Bread:

- Opt for whole-grain versions for added fiber and nutrients.

11. Plant-Based Oils:

- Olive oil, avocado oil, and coconut oil can be used for cooking and dressing.

12. Nutritional Yeast:

- Adds a cheesy flavor and is a good source of B-vitamins, including B12.

13. Plant-Based Protein Sources:

- Beyond tofu and tempeh, explore plant-based protein options like seitan, edamame, and chickpeas.

14. Plant-Based Sweeteners:

- Maple syrup, agave nectar, or date syrup for sweetening dishes.

15. Whole-Grain Flour:

- Use whole-grain flours like whole wheat or almond flour for baking.

16. Plant-Based Condiments:

- Mustard, tahini, soy sauce, and balsamic vinegar for flavor enhancement.

Kitchen Tools and Equipment:

1. Blender:

- Useful for making smoothies, soups, and sauces.

2. Food Processor:

- Great for chopping, slicing, and making homemade dips and spreads.

3. High-Quality Knives:

- A chef's knife, paring knife, and serrated knife for precise cutting.

4. Cutting Boards:

- Multiple boards for fruits, vegetables, and other ingredients to prevent cross-contamination.

5. Non-Stick Cookware:

- Skillets and pots with non-stick surfaces for easy cooking with minimal oil.

6. Baking Sheets and Pans:

- Essential for roasting vegetables, baking, and preparing plant-based desserts.

7. Saucepans and Stockpots:

- For cooking grains, legumes, and preparing soups.

8. Steamer Basket:

- Ideal for preserving the nutrients in vegetables during cooking.

9. Mixing Bowls:

- Various sizes for preparing and mixing ingredients.

10. Measuring Cups and Spoons:

- Accurate measurements for precise cooking and baking.

11. Grater and Zester:

- Useful for adding zest to dishes and grating ingredients like cheese or vegetables.

12. Colander:

- For draining and rinsing beans, lentils, and pasta.

13. Silicone Spatulas and Utensils:

- Gentle on non-stick surfaces and great for stirring and flipping.

14. Bamboo or Wooden Utensils:

- Ideal for mixing and serving without scratching cookware.

15. Food Storage Containers:

- To store prepped ingredients, leftovers, and meals.

16. Vegetable Peeler:

- For peeling and slicing vegetables and fruits.

17. Tongs:

- Handy for flipping items while cooking.

18. Oven Mitts:

- Essential for handling hot pans and trays.

19. Nut Milk Bag or Cheesecloth:

- Useful for making homemade nut milk or straining liquids.

20. Digital Food Thermometer:

- Ensures proper cooking temperatures, especially for plant-based proteins.

Having these essential ingredients and kitchen tools will set you up for success in preparing a wide variety of delicious and nutritious plant-based meals.

CHAPTER 3: NOURISHING RECIPES FOR BONE HEALTH

BREAKFAST BOOSTERS

1. Calcium-Rich Smoothie Bowl

Ingredients:

- 1 cup kale, stems removed
- 1/2 banana, frozen
- 1/2 cup calcium-fortified plant-based milk (like almond or soy)
- 1 tablespoon chia seeds
- 1/4 cup strawberries, sliced
- 1 tablespoon almond butter

Instructions:

- Blend kale, frozen banana, plant-based milk, and chia seeds until smooth.
- Pour into a bowl and top with sliced strawberries and almond butter.

Prep Time: 10 minutes

2. Chickpea Flour Pancakes with Berries

Ingredients:

- 1 cup chickpea flour
- 1 cup water
- 1/2 teaspoon baking powder
- 1/2 teaspoon turmeric
- 1/4 cup blueberries
- 1/4 cup raspberries
- Maple syrup for drizzling

Instructions:

- In a bowl, whisk chickpea flour, water, baking powder, and turmeric until smooth.
- Pour small circles onto a hot, lightly oiled skillet.
- Cook until bubbles form, then flip and cook the other side.
- Top with berries and drizzle with maple syrup.

Prep Time: 15 minutes

3. Vegan Tofu Scramble with Spinach

Ingredients:

- 1/2 block extra-firm tofu, crumbled
- 1 cup spinach, chopped
- 1/2 bell pepper, diced
- 1/4 onion, diced
- 1 clove garlic, minced

- 1/2 teaspoon turmeric
- Salt and pepper to taste
- Whole-grain toast for serving

Instructions:

- Sauté onion and garlic until softened.
- Add bell pepper and cook until slightly tender.
- Stir in crumbled tofu, turmeric, salt, and pepper.
- Add chopped spinach and cook until wilted.
- Serve on whole-grain toast.

Prep Time: 20 minutes

4. Plant-Based Yogurt Parfait

Ingredients:

- 1 cup plant-based yogurt (almond, coconut, or soy)
- 1/2 cup granola
- 1/4 cup mixed berries (blueberries, strawberries)
- 1 tablespoon chia seeds
- 1 tablespoon sliced almonds

Instructions:

- In a glass or bowl, layer plant-based yogurt, granola, mixed berries, chia seeds, and sliced almonds.
- Repeat the layers.

- Top with additional berries and serve.

Prep Time: 10 minutes

5. Almond and Flaxseed Overnight Oats

Ingredients:

- 1/2 cup rolled oats
- 1/2 cup almond milk
- 1 tablespoon almond butter
- 1 tablespoon ground flaxseeds
- 1/2 banana, sliced
- 1/4 cup chopped almonds

Instructions:

- In a jar, combine rolled oats, almond milk, almond butter, and ground flaxseeds.
- Stir well, add sliced banana, and seal the jar.
- Refrigerate overnight.
- Top with chopped almonds before serving.

Prep Time: 5 minutes (plus overnight refrigeration)

6. Spinach and Tomato Breakfast Wrap

Ingredients:

- 1 whole-grain tortilla

- 1 cup fresh spinach
- 1/2 cup cherry tomatoes, halved
- 1/4 cup hummus
- 1/4 avocado, sliced
- Hot sauce (optional)

Instructions:

- Spread hummus on a whole-grain tortilla.
- Layer with fresh spinach, cherry tomatoes, and avocado slices.
- Add hot sauce if desired.
- Roll into a wrap and enjoy.

Prep Time: 10 minutes

7. Berry and Chia Seed Pudding Parfait

Ingredients:

- 1/4 cup chia seeds
- 1 cup plant-based milk
- 1/2 teaspoon vanilla extract
- 1/2 cup mixed berries (strawberries, blueberries)
- 2 tablespoons chopped walnuts

Instructions:

- Mix chia seeds, plant-based milk, and vanilla extract in a jar.

- Refrigerate for at least 2 hours or overnight until it thickens.

- In a glass, layer chia pudding with mixed berries and chopped walnuts.

Prep Time: 5 minutes (plus chilling time)

8. Turmeric and Cinnamon Oatmeal Bowl

Ingredients:

- 1/2 cup rolled oats
- 1 cup water
- 1/2 teaspoon turmeric
- 1/2 teaspoon cinnamon
- 1 tablespoon maple syrup
- 1 tablespoon chopped pecans

Instructions:

- Cook rolled oats with water, turmeric, and cinnamon.
- Stir in maple syrup.
- Top with chopped pecans and serve.

Prep Time: 10 minutes

9. Avocado and Tomato Toast with Hemp Seeds

Ingredients:

- 2 slices whole-grain bread
- 1/2 avocado, mashed
- 1/2 cup cherry tomatoes, sliced
- 1 tablespoon hemp seeds
- Salt and pepper to taste

Instructions:

- Toast whole-grain bread slices.
- Spread mashed avocado on the toast.
- Top with sliced cherry tomatoes.
- Sprinkle hemp seeds, salt, and pepper.

Prep Time: 5 minutes

10. Blueberry and Walnut Muffins

Ingredients:

- 1 1/2 cups whole wheat flour
- 1/2 cup rolled oats
- 1/2 cup chopped walnuts
- 1 teaspoon baking powder
- 1/2 teaspoon baking soda

- 1/4 teaspoon salt
- 1 cup plant-based milk
- 1/4 cup maple syrup
- 1/4 cup applesauce
- 1 teaspoon vanilla extract
- 1 cup blueberries

Instructions:

- Preheat the oven to 350°F (175°C) and line a muffin tin.
- In a bowl, mix flour, oats, chopped walnuts, baking powder, baking soda, and salt.
- In another bowl, whisk plant-based milk, maple syrup, applesauce, and vanilla extract.
- Combine wet and dry ingredients, then fold in blueberries.
- Spoon batter into muffin cups and bake for 20-25 minutes.

Prep Time: 15 minutes

LUNCH RECIPES

1. Quinoa and Vegetable Buddha Bowl

Ingredients:

- 1 cup cooked quinoa
- 1 cup broccoli florets
- 1/2 cup shredded carrots
- 1/2 cup edamame, shelled
- 1/4 cup sliced almonds
- 2 tablespoons tahini
- 1 tablespoon soy sauce
- 1 tablespoon rice vinegar
- 1 teaspoon maple syrup
- Sesame seeds for garnish

Instructions:

- Arrange cooked quinoa, broccoli, shredded carrots, edamame, and sliced almonds in a bowl.
- In a small bowl, whisk together tahini, soy sauce, rice vinegar, and maple syrup.
- Drizzle the dressing over the bowl and garnish with sesame seeds.

Prep Time: 20 minutes

2. Chickpea and Spinach Stuffed Sweet Potatoes

Ingredients:

- 2 medium sweet potatoes, baked
- 1 can (15 oz) chickpeas, drained and rinsed
- 2 cups fresh spinach
- 1/2 red onion, finely chopped
- 1 clove garlic, minced
- 1 teaspoon cumin
- 1/2 teaspoon smoked paprika
- Salt and pepper to taste
- Fresh cilantro for garnish

Instructions:

- In a pan, sauté red onion and garlic until softened.
- Add chickpeas, spinach, cumin, smoked paprika, salt, and pepper.
- Cook until chickpeas are heated through and spinach is wilted.
- Split baked sweet potatoes, and stuff them with the chickpea and spinach mixture.
- Garnish with fresh cilantro.

Prep Time: 30 minutes

3. Vegan Lentil and Vegetable Soup

Ingredients:

- 1 cup green or brown lentils, cooked
- 1 onion, diced
- 2 carrots, sliced
- 2 celery stalks, chopped
- 3 cloves garlic, minced
- 1 can (14 oz) diced tomatoes
- 6 cups vegetable broth
- 1 teaspoon dried thyme
- Salt and pepper to taste
- Fresh parsley for garnish

Instructions:

- In a large pot, sauté onion and garlic until fragrant.
- Add carrots, celery, diced tomatoes, lentils, vegetable broth, thyme, salt, and pepper.
- Bring to a boil, then simmer until vegetables are tender.
- Garnish with fresh parsley before serving.

Prep Time: 40 minutes

4. Mushroom and Spinach Chickpea Stir-Fry

Ingredients:

- 1 can (15 oz) chickpeas, drained and rinsed
- 2 cups mushrooms, sliced
- 3 cups fresh spinach
- 1 bell pepper, sliced
- 1/4 cup low-sodium soy sauce
- 1 tablespoon maple syrup
- 1 tablespoon sesame oil
- 1 teaspoon grated ginger
- Brown rice for serving

Instructions:

- In a wok or pan, sauté mushrooms until they release their moisture.
- Add chickpeas, fresh spinach, bell pepper, soy sauce, maple syrup, sesame oil, and grated ginger.
- Stir-fry until the vegetables are tender.
- Serve over brown rice.

Prep Time: 25 minutes

5. Stuffed Bell Peppers with Quinoa and Black Beans

Ingredients:

- 4 bell peppers, halved
- 1 cup cooked quinoa
- 1 can (15 oz) black beans, drained and rinsed
- 1 cup corn kernels (fresh or frozen)
- 1 cup diced tomatoes
- 1 teaspoon cumin
- 1/2 teaspoon chili powder
- Salt and pepper to taste
- Guacamole for topping

Instructions:

- Preheat the oven to 375°F (190°C).
- In a bowl, mix cooked quinoa, black beans, corn, diced tomatoes, cumin, chili powder, salt, and pepper.
- Stuff halved bell peppers with the quinoa mixture.
- Bake in the oven until peppers are tender.
- Top with guacamole before serving.

Prep Time: 35 minutes

6. Chia Seed and Mixed Berry Salad

Ingredients:

- 2 cups mixed greens (spinach, arugula, kale)
- 1 cup mixed berries (blueberries, strawberries, raspberries)
- 2 tablespoons chia seeds
- 1/4 cup walnuts, chopped
- Balsamic vinaigrette dressing

Instructions:

- In a bowl, toss mixed greens, mixed berries, chia seeds, and chopped walnuts.
- Drizzle with balsamic vinaigrette dressing and toss to coat.

Prep Time: 10 minutes

7. Roasted Vegetable Quinoa Bowl

Ingredients:

- 1 cup cooked quinoa
- 1 cup broccoli florets
- 1/2 cup cherry tomatoes, halved
- 1/2 cup carrots, sliced
- 1/2 cup red bell pepper, sliced

- 2 tablespoons olive oil
- 1 teaspoon dried rosemary
- Salt and pepper to taste
- Lemon tahini dressing for drizzling

Instructions:

- Preheat the oven to 400°F (200°C).
- Toss broccoli, cherry tomatoes, carrots, and red bell pepper with olive oil, dried rosemary, salt, and pepper.
- Roast in the oven until vegetables are tender.
- Arrange cooked quinoa in a bowl, top with roasted vegetables, and drizzle with lemon tahini dressing.

Prep Time: 30 minutes

8. Vegan Caesar Salad with Chickpea Croutons

Ingredients:

- 1 head romaine lettuce, chopped
- 1 cup cherry tomatoes, halved
- 1/4 cup red onion, thinly sliced
- **For Dressing:** 1/4 cup tahini, 2 tablespoons nutritional yeast, 1 tablespoon lemon juice, 1 clove garlic, minced, salt, and pepper to taste

- **For Chickpea Croutons:** 1 can (15 oz) chickpeas, drained, 1 tablespoon olive oil, 1 teaspoon garlic powder, 1 teaspoon smoked paprika, salt to taste

Instructions:

- Preheat the oven to 400°F (200°C).
- Toss chickpeas with olive oil, garlic powder, smoked paprika, and salt.
- Roast in the oven until crispy.
- In a large bowl, combine chopped romaine lettuce, cherry tomatoes, and sliced red onion.
- In a small bowl, whisk together tahini, nutritional yeast, lemon juice, minced garlic, salt, and pepper.
- Pour the dressing over the salad and top with chickpea croutons.

Prep Time: 25 minutes

9. Lemon Herb Tofu Skewers with Quinoa

Ingredients:

- 1 block extra-firm tofu, cubed
- 2 tablespoons lemon juice
- 2 tablespoons olive oil
- 1 teaspoon dried oregano

- 1 teaspoon dried thyme
- Salt and pepper to taste
- Quinoa for serving
- Cherry tomatoes for skewering

Instructions:

- In a bowl, marinate tofu cubes in lemon juice, olive oil, oregano, thyme, salt, and pepper.
- Thread marinated tofu and cherry tomatoes onto skewers.
- Grill or bake until tofu is golden brown.
- Serve over a bed of quinoa.

Prep Time: 30 minutes (including marinating time)

10. Cauliflower and Lentil Curry

Ingredients:

- 1 cup green or brown lentils, cooked
- 1 head cauliflower, cut into florets
- 1 can (14 oz) coconut milk
- 1 onion, diced
- 3 cloves garlic, minced
- 1 tablespoon curry powder
- 1 teaspoon turmeric
- Salt and pepper to taste

- Fresh cilantro for garnish

- Brown rice for serving

Instructions:

- In a pot, sauté onion and garlic until softened.
- Add cauliflower florets, cooked lentils, coconut milk, curry powder, turmeric, salt, and pepper.
- Simmer until cauliflower is tender.
- Garnish with fresh cilantro and serve over brown rice.

Prep Time: 40 minutes

1. Stuffed Bell Peppers with Quinoa and Black Beans

Ingredients:

- 4 bell peppers, halved
- 1 cup cooked quinoa
- 1 can (15 oz) black beans, drained and rinsed
- 1 cup corn kernels (fresh or frozen)
- 1 cup diced tomatoes
- 1 teaspoon cumin
- 1/2 teaspoon chili powder
- Salt and pepper to taste
- Guacamole for topping

Instructions:

- Preheat the oven to 375°F (190°C).
- In a bowl, mix cooked quinoa, black beans, corn, diced tomatoes, cumin, chili powder, salt, and pepper.
- Stuff halved bell peppers with the quinoa mixture.
- Bake in the oven until peppers are tender.
- Top with guacamole before serving.

Prep Time: 35 minutes

2. Chickpea and Spinach Curry

Ingredients:

- 1 can (15 oz) chickpeas, drained and rinsed
- 2 cups fresh spinach
- 1 onion, finely chopped
- 3 cloves garlic, minced
- 1 can (14 oz) diced tomatoes
- 1 can (14 oz) coconut milk
- 2 tablespoons curry powder
- 1 teaspoon ground cumin
- 1 teaspoon ground coriander
- Salt and pepper to taste
- Fresh cilantro for garnish
- Brown rice for serving

Instructions:

- In a pan, sauté onion and garlic until softened.
- Add chickpeas, diced tomatoes, coconut milk, curry powder, cumin, coriander, salt, and pepper.
- Simmer until the sauce thickens and flavors meld.
- Stir in fresh spinach until wilted.
- Garnish with fresh cilantro and serve over brown rice.

Prep Time: 40 minutes

3. Vegan Lentil Loaf

Ingredients:

- 2 cups cooked green or brown lentils
- 1 cup rolled oats
- 1 onion, finely chopped
- 2 carrots, grated
- 1/2 cup tomato sauce
- 2 tablespoons soy sauce
- 1 teaspoon dried thyme
- 1 teaspoon dried rosemary
- Salt and pepper to taste
- **For Glaze:** 1/4 cup ketchup, 1 tablespoon maple syrup, 1 teaspoon Dijon mustard

Instructions:

- Preheat the oven to 350°F (175°C).
- In a food processor, blend cooked lentils, rolled oats, onion, carrots, tomato sauce, soy sauce, thyme, rosemary, salt, and pepper.
- Transfer the mixture to a loaf pan.
- In a small bowl, mix ketchup, maple syrup, and Dijon mustard for the glaze.
- Spread the glaze over the lentil loaf.
- Bake in the oven for 40-45 minutes.

Prep Time: 50 minutes

4. Spaghetti Squash Primavera

Ingredients:

- 1 medium spaghetti squash, halved and seeds removed
- 1 cup cherry tomatoes, halved
- 1 cup broccoli florets
- 1/2 red bell pepper, sliced
- 2 cloves garlic, minced
- 2 tablespoons olive oil
- 1 teaspoon dried oregano
- Salt and pepper to taste
- Fresh basil for garnish

Instructions:

- Preheat the oven to 400°F (200°C).
- Place spaghetti squash halves on a baking sheet, cut side up.
- In a bowl, toss cherry tomatoes, broccoli, red bell pepper, garlic, olive oil, oregano, salt, and pepper.
- Spread the vegetable mixture around the spaghetti squash.
- Roast in the oven until squash is tender.

- Use a fork to scrape the spaghetti-like strands from the squash.
- Serve with roasted vegetables and garnish with fresh basil.

Prep Time: 45 minutes

5. Mushroom and Lentil Shepherd's Pie

Ingredients:

- 2 cups cooked green or brown lentils
- 1 cup mushrooms, chopped
- 1 onion, diced
- 2 carrots, diced
- 1 cup peas (fresh or frozen)
- 2 cloves garlic, minced
- 1 cup vegetable broth
- 2 tablespoons tomato paste
- 1 teaspoon dried thyme
- Mashed sweet potatoes for topping

Instructions:

- Preheat the oven to 375°F (190°C).
- In a pan, sauté onion and garlic until softened.
- Add mushrooms, carrots, peas, lentils, vegetable broth, tomato paste, and thyme.

- Simmer until the mixture thickens.
- Transfer the lentil mixture to a baking dish.
- Top with mashed sweet potatoes.
- Bake in the oven until the top is golden brown.

Prep Time: 50 minutes

6. Veggie and Tofu Stir-Fry

Ingredients:

- 1 block extra-firm tofu, cubed
- 2 cups broccoli florets
- 1 bell pepper, sliced
- 1 carrot, julienned
- 1 cup snap peas
- 3 tablespoons soy sauce
- 1 tablespoon sesame oil
- 1 tablespoon maple syrup
- 1 teaspoon grated ginger
- 2 cloves garlic, minced
- Brown rice for serving

Instructions:

- In a wok or pan, sauté tofu cubes until golden brown.
- Add broccoli, bell pepper, carrot, and snap peas.

- In a bowl, whisk together soy sauce, sesame oil, maple syrup, grated ginger, and minced garlic.
- Pour the sauce over the vegetables and tofu. Stir-fry until vegetables are tender.
- Serve over brown rice.

Prep Time: 30 minutes

7. Stuffed Acorn Squash with Quinoa and Cranberries

Ingredients:

- 2 acorn squash, halved and seeds removed
- 1 cup cooked quinoa
- 1/2 cup dried cranberries
- 1/4 cup chopped pecans
- 2 tablespoons maple syrup
- 1 teaspoon cinnamon
- Salt and pepper to taste
- Fresh parsley for garnish

Instructions:

- Preheat the oven to 400°F (200°C).
- Place acorn squash halves on a baking sheet, cut side up.

* In a bowl, mix cooked quinoa, dried cranberries, chopped pecans, maple syrup, cinnamon, salt, and pepper.
* Stuff each acorn squash half with the quinoa mixture.
* Bake in the oven until squash is tender.
* Garnish with fresh parsley before serving.

Prep Time: 45 minutes

8. Chickpea and Sweet Potato Curry

Ingredients:

* 1 can (15 oz) chickpeas, drained and rinsed
* 2 sweet potatoes, peeled and diced
* 1 can (14 oz) coconut milk
* 1 onion, diced
* 3 cloves garlic, minced
* 1 tablespoon curry powder
* 1 teaspoon ground cumin
* 1 teaspoon ground coriander
* Salt and pepper to taste
* Fresh cilantro for garnish
* Quinoa or brown rice for serving

Instructions:

* In a pot, sauté onion and garlic until softened.

- Add sweet potatoes, chickpeas, coconut milk, curry powder, cumin, coriander, salt, and pepper.
- Simmer until sweet potatoes are tender.
- Garnish with fresh cilantro and serve over quinoa or brown rice.

Prep Time: 40 minutes

9. Lemon Garlic Roasted Brussels Sprouts and Chickpeas

Ingredients:

- 2 cups Brussels sprouts, halved
- 1 can (15 oz) chickpeas, drained and rinsed
- 2 tablespoons olive oil
- 2 cloves garlic, minced
- 1 teaspoon lemon zest
- 1 tablespoon lemon juice
- Salt and pepper to taste

Instructions:

- Preheat the oven to 400°F (200°C).
- Toss Brussels sprouts and chickpeas with olive oil, minced garlic, lemon zest, lemon juice, salt, and pepper.
- Spread on a baking sheet.

- Roast in the oven until Brussels sprouts are crispy and chickpeas are golden brown.

Prep Time: 30 minutes

10. Cauliflower and Chickpea Coconut Curry

Ingredients:

- 1 can (15 oz) chickpeas, drained and rinsed
- 1 head cauliflower, cut into florets
- 1 can (14 oz) coconut milk
- 1 onion, diced
- 3 cloves garlic, minced
- 1 tablespoon curry powder
- 1 teaspoon ground turmeric
- Salt and pepper to taste
- Fresh cilantro for garnish
- Basmati rice for serving

Instructions:

- In a pot, sauté onion and garlic until softened.
- Add chickpeas, cauliflower florets, coconut milk, curry powder, turmeric, salt, and pepper.
- Simmer until cauliflower is tender.

- Garnish with fresh cilantro and serve over basmati rice.

Prep Time: 40 minutes

SNACKS AND APPETIZERS

1. Roasted Chickpeas with Turmeric and Cumin

Ingredients:

- 1 can (15 oz) chickpeas, drained and rinsed
- 1 tablespoon olive oil
- 1/2 teaspoon turmeric
- 1/2 teaspoon cumin
- 1/2 teaspoon smoked paprika
- Salt to taste

Instructions:

- Preheat the oven to 400°F (200°C).
- Pat chickpeas dry and toss with olive oil, turmeric, cumin, smoked paprika, and salt.
- Spread on a baking sheet and roast until crispy, shaking the pan occasionally.
- Let cool before serving.

Prep Time: 30 minutes

2. Guacamole with Veggie Sticks

Ingredients:

- 3 ripe avocados
- 1 tomato, diced
- 1/4 cup red onion, finely chopped
- 1 clove garlic, minced
- 1 lime, juiced
- Salt and pepper to taste
- Carrot and cucumber sticks for dipping

Instructions:

- Mash avocados in a bowl.
- Add diced tomato, red onion, minced garlic, lime juice, salt, and pepper. Mix well.
- Serve with carrot and cucumber sticks.

Prep Time: 15 minutes

3. Sesame Kale Chips

Ingredients:

- 1 bunch kale, stems removed and torn into bite-sized pieces
- 1 tablespoon sesame oil
- 1 tablespoon soy sauce
- 1 tablespoon nutritional yeast
- 1 teaspoon sesame seeds

Instructions:

- Preheat the oven to 350°F (175°C).
- In a bowl, toss kale with sesame oil, soy sauce, nutritional yeast, and sesame seeds.
- Spread on a baking sheet and bake until crispy.

Prep Time: 20 minutes

4. Hummus and Veggie Pinwheels

Ingredients:

- Whole-grain tortillas
- 1 cup hummus
- 1/2 cucumber, thinly sliced
- 1/2 bell pepper, thinly sliced
- 1/4 cup baby spinach leaves

Instructions:

- Spread a layer of hummus on each tortilla.
- Layer cucumber, bell pepper, and spinach leaves.
- Roll tightly and slice into pinwheels.

Prep Time: 15 minutes

5. Tomato Basil Bruschetta

Ingredients:

- 4 tomatoes, diced
- 1/4 cup fresh basil, chopped
- 2 cloves garlic, minced
- 1 tablespoon balsamic vinegar
- 2 tablespoons olive oil
- Salt and pepper to taste
- Whole-grain baguette slices for serving

Instructions:

- In a bowl, combine diced tomatoes, chopped basil, minced garlic, balsamic vinegar, olive oil, salt, and pepper.
- Let the mixture sit for flavors to meld.
- Serve on whole-grain baguette slices.

Prep Time: 15 minutes

6. Edamame and Avocado Dip

Ingredients:

- 1 cup edamame, shelled and cooked
- 1 ripe avocado
- 2 tablespoons lime juice
- 1 clove garlic, minced
- Salt and pepper to taste
- Whole-grain pita chips for dipping

Instructions:

- In a blender or food processor, combine edamame, avocado, lime juice, minced garlic, salt, and pepper.
- Blend until smooth.
- Serve with whole-grain pita chips.

Prep Time: 15 minutes

7. Cucumber and Dill Yogurt Bites

Ingredients:

- 1 cucumber, sliced
- 1 cup plant-based yogurt
- 1 tablespoon fresh dill, chopped
- 1 teaspoon lemon zest
- Salt and pepper to taste

Instructions:

- In a bowl, mix plant-based yogurt, chopped dill, lemon zest, salt, and pepper.
- Top cucumber slices with the yogurt mixture.

Prep Time: 10 minutes

8. Sweet Potato and Black Bean Quesadillas

Ingredients:

- Whole-grain tortillas
- 1 cup sweet potato, cooked and mashed
- 1 can (15 oz) black beans, drained and rinsed
- 1/2 cup corn kernels (fresh or frozen)
- 1 teaspoon cumin
- 1/2 teaspoon chili powder
- Guacamole for topping

Instructions:

- On a tortilla, spread a layer of mashed sweet potato.
- Top with black beans, corn, cumin, and chili powder.
- Place another tortilla on top and cook in a skillet until golden brown.
- Slice into wedges and serve with guacamole.

Prep Time: 25 minutes

9. Berry and Almond Energy Bites

Ingredients:

- 1 cup mixed berries (blueberries, raspberries)
- 1 cup rolled oats

- 1/2 cup almond butter
- 1/4 cup chia seeds
- 1/4 cup maple syrup
- 1/2 cup chopped almonds

Instructions:

- In a food processor, blend mixed berries, rolled oats, almond butter, chia seeds, and maple syrup until smooth.
- Transfer the mixture to a bowl and fold in chopped almonds.
- Form into bite-sized balls and refrigerate until firm.

Prep Time: 20 minutes

10. Stuffed Mini Peppers with Quinoa and Salsa

Ingredients:

- Mini bell peppers, halved and seeds removed
- 1 cup cooked quinoa
- 1/2 cup black beans, drained and rinsed
- 1/2 cup corn kernels (fresh or frozen)
- 1/2 cup cherry tomatoes, diced
- 1/4 cup red onion, finely chopped
- Fresh cilantro for garnish

Instructions:

- In a bowl, mix cooked quinoa, black beans, corn, cherry tomatoes, and red onion.
- Spoon the quinoa mixture into halved mini peppers.
- Garnish with fresh cilantro.

Prep Time: 20 minutes

DESSERT RECIPES

1. Mixed Berry Chia Pudding

Ingredients:

- 1/4 cup chia seeds
- 1 cup plant-based milk (almond, soy, or coconut)
- 1 tablespoon maple syrup
- 1 teaspoon vanilla extract
- Mixed berries for topping

Instructions:

- In a bowl, mix chia seeds, plant-based milk, maple syrup, and vanilla extract.
- Refrigerate for at least 2 hours or overnight until the mixture thickens.
- Top with mixed berries before serving.

Prep Time: 5 minutes + chilling time

2. Chocolate Avocado Mousse

Ingredients:

- 2 ripe avocados
- 1/4 cup cocoa powder
- 1/4 cup maple syrup
- 1 teaspoon vanilla extract

- Pinch of salt

- Fresh berries for garnish

Instructions:

- In a blender, combine avocados, cocoa powder, maple syrup, vanilla extract, and salt.

- Blend until smooth and creamy.

- Refrigerate for at least 1 hour before serving.

- Garnish with fresh berries.

Prep Time: 10 minutes + chilling time

3. Banana Oat Cookies

Ingredients:

- 2 ripe bananas, mashed

- 1 cup rolled oats

- 1/4 cup chopped nuts (walnuts or almonds)

- 1/4 cup raisins

- 1 teaspoon vanilla extract

- 1/2 teaspoon cinnamon

Instructions:

- Preheat the oven to 350°F (175°C).

- In a bowl, mix mashed bananas, rolled oats, chopped nuts, raisins, vanilla extract, and cinnamon.

- Drop spoonfuls of the mixture onto a baking sheet.
- Bake for 12-15 minutes or until golden brown.

Prep Time: 10 minutes + baking time

4. Coconut and Berry Parfait

Ingredients:

- 1 cup coconut yogurt
- 1/2 cup granola
- Mixed berries (blueberries, strawberries, raspberries)
- 1 tablespoon shredded coconut

Instructions:

- In a glass or bowl, layer coconut yogurt, granola, and mixed berries.
- Repeat the layers.
- Top with shredded coconut before serving.

Prep Time: 5 minutes

5. Pumpkin Spice Energy Bites

Ingredients:

- 1 cup rolled oats
- 1/2 cup pumpkin puree
- 1/4 cup almond butter

- 1/4 cup maple syrup
- 1 teaspoon pumpkin spice
- 1/4 cup chopped pecans

Instructions:

- In a bowl, mix rolled oats, pumpkin puree, almond butter, maple syrup, pumpkin spice, and chopped pecans.
- Form the mixture into bite-sized balls.
- Refrigerate until firm before serving.

Prep Time: 15 minutes + chilling time

6. Date and Nut Bars

Ingredients:

- 1 cup dates, pitted
- 1 cup mixed nuts (almonds, walnuts, cashews)
- 1/4 cup shredded coconut
- 1/4 cup cacao powder
- Pinch of salt

Instructions:

- In a food processor, blend dates, mixed nuts, shredded coconut, cacao powder, and salt until a sticky dough forms.

- Press the mixture into a lined pan.
- Refrigerate for at least 1 hour before cutting into bars.

Prep Time: 15 minutes + chilling time

7. Baked Apples with Cinnamon

Ingredients:

- 4 apples, cored and halved
- 2 tablespoons maple syrup
- 1 teaspoon cinnamon
- Chopped nuts for topping

Instructions:

- Preheat the oven to 375°F (190°C).
- Place apple halves on a baking sheet.
- Drizzle with maple syrup and sprinkle with cinnamon.
- Bake until apples are tender.
- Top with chopped nuts before serving.

Prep Time: 15 minutes + baking time

8. Chocolate-Dipped Strawberries

Ingredients:

- 1 cup dark chocolate chips
- 1 tablespoon coconut oil

- Fresh strawberries

Instructions:

- In a bowl, melt dark chocolate chips and coconut oil together.
- Dip each strawberry into the melted chocolate, coating it halfway.
- Place on a parchment-lined tray.
- Refrigerate until the chocolate is set.

Prep Time: 15 minutes + chilling time

9. Mango Sorbet

Ingredients:

- 2 cups frozen mango chunks
- 1/4 cup coconut water
- 1 tablespoon lime juice
- Mint leaves for garnish

Instructions:

- In a blender, blend frozen mango chunks, coconut water, and lime juice until smooth.
- Transfer to a dish and freeze for at least 2 hours.
- Scoop into bowls and garnish with mint leaves.

Prep Time: 10 minutes + freezing time

10. Almond and Berry Popsicles

Ingredients:

- 1 cup almond milk
- 1/2 cup mixed berries (blueberries, raspberries)
- 1 tablespoon maple syrup
- 1/4 cup sliced almonds

Instructions:

- In a blender, blend almond milk, mixed berries, and maple syrup until smooth.
- Stir in sliced almonds.
- Pour the mixture into popsicle molds and freeze until solid.

Prep Time: 10 minutes + freezing time

SMOOTHIES AND BEVERAGES

1. Green Calcium Boost Smoothie

Ingredients:

- 1 cup kale, stems removed
- 1/2 cup broccoli florets
- 1 ripe banana
- 1/2 cup orange juice
- 1 tablespoon chia seeds
- 1 cup plant-based milk (almond, soy, or oat)

Instructions:

- In a blender, combine kale, broccoli, banana, orange juice, chia seeds, and plant-based milk.
- Blend until smooth.
- Pour into a glass and enjoy.

Prep Time: 5 minutes

2. Berry Bliss Calcium Smoothie

Ingredients:

- 1 cup mixed berries (blueberries, strawberries, raspberries)
- 1/2 cup silken tofu
- 1 tablespoon almond butter

- 1 tablespoon flaxseeds
- 1 cup fortified plant-based milk (such as almond or soy)

Instructions:

- Blend mixed berries, silken tofu, almond butter, flaxseeds, and plant-based milk until creamy.
- Pour into a glass and serve.

Prep Time: 5 minutes

3. Tropical Vitamin C Smoothie

Ingredients:

- 1 cup pineapple chunks
- 1/2 cup mango chunks
- 1/2 cup kale, stems removed
- 1 tablespoon hemp seeds
- 1 cup coconut water

Instructions:

- In a blender, combine pineapple chunks, mango chunks, kale, hemp seeds, and coconut water.
- Blend until smooth.
- Pour into a glass and enjoy.

Prep Time: 5 minutes

4. Golden Turmeric Latte

Ingredients:

- 1 cup unsweetened almond milk
- 1 teaspoon ground turmeric
- 1/2 teaspoon ground cinnamon
- 1/4 teaspoon ground ginger
- 1 tablespoon maple syrup
- Pinch of black pepper

Instructions:

- In a saucepan, heat almond milk, turmeric, cinnamon, ginger, maple syrup, and black pepper.
- Whisk until well combined and heated through.
- Pour into a mug and enjoy.

Prep Time: 5 minutes

5. Citrus Vitamin D Booster Smoothie

Ingredients:

- 1 orange, peeled and segmented
- 1/2 cup mango chunks
- 1/2 cup fortified orange juice
- 1 tablespoon chia seeds
- 1 cup plant-based yogurt

**Instructions:**

- Blend orange segments, mango chunks, fortified orange juice, chia seeds, and plant-based yogurt until smooth.
- Pour into a glass and serve.

**Prep Time: 5 minutes**

6. Calcium-Rich Chocolate Almond Smoothie

**Ingredients:**

- 1 cup fortified chocolate almond milk
- 1/2 cup silken tofu
- 1 tablespoon almond butter
- 1 tablespoon cacao powder
- 1 tablespoon flaxseeds

**Instructions:**

- Blend chocolate almond milk, silken tofu, almond butter, cacao powder, and flaxseeds until creamy.
- Pour into a glass and enjoy.

**Prep Time: 5 minutes**

7. Antioxidant Berry Iced Tea

Ingredients:

- 1 cup mixed berries (blueberries, raspberries)
- 1 tablespoon hibiscus tea leaves
- 1 tablespoon maple syrup
- 1 lemon, sliced
- 4 cups cold water

Instructions:

- In a pitcher, muddle mixed berries with hibiscus tea leaves and maple syrup.
- Add lemon slices and cold water.
- Stir well and refrigerate for at least 2 hours.
- Strain before serving over ice.

Prep Time: 5 minutes + chilling time

8. Almond and Date Protein Smoothie

Ingredients:

- 1 cup almond milk
- 1/2 cup silken tofu
- 2 dates, pitted
- 1 tablespoon almond butter
- 1 tablespoon hemp seeds

Instructions:

- Blend almond milk, silken tofu, dates, almond butter, and hemp seeds until smooth.
- Pour into a glass and enjoy.

Prep Time: 5 minutes

9. Minty Avocado Green Tea

Ingredients:

- 1 cup brewed green tea, chilled
- 1/2 avocado, peeled and pitted
- 1 tablespoon fresh mint leaves
- 1 tablespoon agave syrup
- Ice cubes

Instructions:

- In a blender, combine chilled green tea, avocado, mint leaves, and agave syrup.
- Blend until smooth.
- Pour over ice and serve.

Prep Time: 5 minutes

10. Pomegranate and Walnut Smoothie

Ingredients:

- 1 cup pomegranate seeds
- 1/4 cup walnuts
- 1/2 cup spinach leaves
- 1 tablespoon chia seeds
- 1 cup coconut water

Instructions:

- Blend pomegranate seeds, walnuts, spinach leaves, chia seeds, and coconut water until smooth.
- Pour into a glass and enjoy.

Prep Time: 5 minutes

CHAPTER 4: BONE-BOOSTING TIPS AND TRICKS

Incorporating Calcium-Rich Foods

1. Leafy Greens:

- **Sources:** Kale, bok choy, collard greens, turnip greens, broccoli
- **Incorporation:** Add kale or spinach to smoothies, make a hearty salad with mixed greens, or sauté greens as a side dish.

2. Tofu and Tempeh:

- **Sources:** Firm tofu, tempeh
- **Incorporation:** Grill or stir-fry tofu and tempeh, add them to curries or salads, or use them in plant-based sandwiches and wraps.

3. Fortified Plant Milks:

- **Sources:** Fortified almond milk, soy milk, oat milk
- **Incorporation:** Use fortified plant milk in your morning cereal, oatmeal, or coffee. It can also be used in cooking and baking.

4. Almonds:

- **Sources:** Almonds
- **Incorporation:** Snack on almonds, add them to salads, sprinkle chopped almonds on yogurt or cereal, or use almond butter as a spread.

5. Chia Seeds:

- **Sources:** Chia seeds
- **Incorporation:** Make chia pudding by combining chia seeds with plant milk and letting it sit overnight. Add fruits for sweetness and flavor.

6. Legumes:

- **Sources:** Chickpeas, black beans, lentils
- **Incorporation:** Include legumes in salads, soups, stews, and curries. Make hummus with chickpeas for a tasty dip.

7. Fortified Breakfast Cereals:

- **Sources:** Fortified cereals
- **Incorporation:** Enjoy a bowl of fortified cereal with fortified plant milk for a quick and convenient calcium boost.

8. Sesame Seeds and Tahini:

- **Sources:** Sesame seeds, tahini

- **Incorporation:** Sprinkle sesame seeds on salads or stir-fries, and use tahini in dressings, dips, or as a spread on whole-grain bread.

9. Oranges:

- **Sources:** Oranges
- **Incorporation:** Snack on fresh oranges, make a citrusy salad, or squeeze fresh orange juice to accompany your meals.

10. Dried Fruits:

- **Sources:** Figs, apricots
- **Incorporation:** Snack on dried figs and apricots or add them to cereals, salads, or homemade trail mixes.

Vitamin D and Sunlight Exposure

The Importance of Vitamin D for Bone Health:

1. Calcium Absorption:

- **Role:** Vitamin D is crucial for the absorption of calcium in the intestines.
- **Significance:** Adequate calcium absorption is essential for maintaining strong and healthy bones.

2. Bone Mineralization:

- **Role:** Vitamin D promotes bone mineralization, helping to incorporate minerals like calcium and phosphorus into the bone matrix.
- **Significance:** This process contributes to bone strength and density.

3. Regulation of Calcium and Phosphorus:

- **Role:** Vitamin D helps regulate calcium and phosphorus levels in the blood.
- **Significance:** Maintaining optimal blood levels of these minerals is vital for various physiological functions, including nerve transmission and muscle function.

4. Prevention of Rickets and Osteomalacia:

- **Role:** Adequate vitamin D prevents conditions like rickets in children and osteomalacia in adults, which are characterized by weakened and soft bones.
- **Significance:** Ensuring sufficient vitamin D levels is crucial for preventing these bone disorders.

5. Support for Bone Remodeling:

- **Role:** Vitamin D supports the process of bone remodeling, where old bone tissue is replaced by new bone tissue.

- **Significance:** This continuous remodeling process is essential for maintaining bone strength and adapting to changes in physical activity levels.

Safe Sun Exposure and Alternatives:

1. Sun Exposure:

Duration and Timing:

- **Recommendation:** Aim for 10-30 minutes of sunlight exposure to large areas of the skin, such as arms, legs, or back, at least twice a week.

- **Best Time:** Sun exposure is most effective during midday when the sun is at its highest point in the sky.

2. Sunscreen Use:

- **Importance:** While sunscreen protects the skin from harmful UV rays, it can also inhibit vitamin D synthesis.

- **Balance:** Find a balance between sun protection and vitamin D synthesis. Consider exposing unprotected skin for a short duration before applying sunscreen.

3. Alternative Sources of Vitamin D:

Dietary Sources:

- Include vitamin D-rich foods in your diet, such as fatty fish (salmon, mackerel), fortified plant milks, fortified orange juice, and mushrooms exposed to sunlight.

Supplements:

- Consult with a healthcare professional to determine if vitamin D supplements are necessary, especially if you have limited sun exposure or specific health conditions.

4. UVB Lamps:

- **Usage:** UVB lamps or bulbs designed for vitamin D production can be used under controlled conditions.

- **Caution:** Use with caution and consult with a healthcare professional to ensure proper usage and minimize risks.

5. Regular Testing:

- **Importance:** Periodically check your vitamin D levels through blood tests.
- **Guidance:** Consult with a healthcare professional to interpret results and adjust your sun exposure or supplementation accordingly.

6. Fortified Foods:

- **Options:** Include fortified foods like cereals, plant milks, and nutritional yeast in your diet.
- **Convenience:** Fortified foods provide a convenient way to ensure adequate vitamin D intake, especially in plant-based diets.

7. Professional Guidance:

- **Individualized Recommendations:** Consult with a healthcare professional or a registered dietitian for personalized recommendations based on your specific health status, dietary habits, and lifestyle.

Balancing Nutrients for Optimal Absorption

Combining Foods for Maximum Nutrient Bioavailability:

1. Vitamin C and Iron:

- **Combination:** Pair iron-rich plant foods with vitamin C-rich foods.
- **Example:** Add bell peppers, citrus fruits, or tomatoes to iron-rich dishes like lentils, beans, or spinach.
- **Benefit:** Vitamin C enhances the absorption of non-heme iron found in plant-based sources.

2. Iron and Vitamin A:

- **Combination:** Combine iron-rich foods with those high in vitamin A.
- **Example:** Pair sweet potatoes, carrots, or dark leafy greens with beans or lentils.

- **Benefit:** Vitamin A supports the utilization of iron for various bodily functions.

3. Iron and Vitamin B12:

- **Combination:** Consume iron-rich plant foods along with vitamin B12 sources.

- **Example:** Lentils or fortified cereals with nutritional yeast or fortified plant milk.

- **Benefit:** Vitamin B12 supports iron absorption and helps prevent anemia.

4. Calcium and Vitamin D:

- **Combination:** Consume calcium-rich plant foods with vitamin D sources.

- **Example:** Fortified plant milk or fortified orange juice with exposure to sunlight for vitamin D.

- **Benefit:** Vitamin D enhances calcium absorption, promoting bone health.

5. Calcium and Magnesium:

- **Combination:** Include magnesium-rich foods with calcium sources.
- **Example:** Combine almonds, spinach, or whole grains with calcium-rich foods like fortified plant milk.
- **Benefit:** Balanced magnesium levels support optimal calcium absorption.

6. Protein and Zinc:

- **Combination:** Pair plant-based protein sources with zinc-rich foods.
- **Example:** Lentils or chickpeas with seeds like pumpkin seeds.
- **Benefit:** Adequate zinc supports protein synthesis and immune function.

7. Vitamin K and Healthy Fats:

- **Combination:** Include vitamin K-rich greens with healthy fats.
- **Example:** Kale or spinach salad with an olive oil dressing.

- **Benefit:** Healthy fats aid in the absorption of fat-soluble vitamins, including vitamin K.

Understanding Plant-Based Iron Sources:

1. Non-Heme Iron:

- **Sources:** Found in plant foods such as legumes (lentils, beans), tofu, fortified cereals, nuts, seeds, and leafy greens (spinach, kale).
- **Enhancement:** Combine non-heme iron sources with vitamin C-rich foods to improve absorption.

2. Enhancers of Iron Absorption:

- **Vitamin C:** Enhances non-heme iron absorption. Include citrus fruits, strawberries, bell peppers, and tomatoes.
- **Beta-Carotene:** Found in carrots, sweet potatoes, and dark leafy greens, it supports iron utilization.
- **Fermentable Foods:** Some fermented foods may enhance iron absorption.

3. Inhibitors of Iron Absorption:

- **Phytates:** Present in some plant foods, they can inhibit iron absorption. Soaking, fermenting, or cooking can reduce phytate levels.
- **Tannins:** Found in tea and coffee, they may hinder iron absorption. Consider consuming these beverages between meals.

4. Iron-Rich Plant Foods:

- **Legumes:** Lentils, chickpeas, black beans.
- **Tofu and Tempeh:** Excellent plant-based protein sources containing iron.
- **Nuts and Seeds:** Almonds, pumpkin seeds, hemp seeds.
- **Leafy Greens:** Spinach, kale, collard greens.

5. Pairing Iron-Rich Foods:

- **Example Meal:** Lentil salad with spinach, cherry tomatoes, bell peppers, and a lemon vinaigrette.
- **Tip:** Include a vitamin C-rich fruit as dessert or a snack.

6. Fortified Foods:

- **Options:** Choose fortified cereals, plant milk, and nutritional yeast to increase iron intake.
- **Check Labels:** Look for products fortified with iron, especially if following a strict plant-based diet.

CHAPTER 5: LIFESTYLE PRACTICES FOR STRONGER BONES

Physical Activity and Bone Health

Physical activity plays a crucial role in maintaining bone health and preventing conditions like osteoporosis. Here are key aspects of how exercise impacts bone health:

1. Weight-Bearing Exercise:

- **Definition:** Weight-bearing exercises involve activities that force you to work against gravity.
- **Impact:** These exercises, such as walking, running, dancing, and strength training, help stimulate bone-forming cells and improve bone density.

2. Strength Training:

- **Definition:** Strength or resistance training involves lifting weights or using resistance to build muscle strength.
- **Impact:** It not only increases muscle mass but also stimulates the bones to become denser and stronger. Focus on exercises targeting major muscle groups.

3. High-Impact vs. Low-Impact Exercise:

- **High-Impact:** Activities like running, jumping, and aerobics can help build bone density but may put stress on joints.

- **Low-Impact:** Exercises like walking, swimming, or cycling are gentler on joints while still promoting bone health.

4. Balance and Stability Exercises:

- **Definition:** Balance exercises help improve stability and reduce the risk of falls.

- **Impact:** Incorporating activities like yoga or tai chi can enhance balance and coordination, reducing the likelihood of fractures.

5. Frequency and Duration:

- **Recommendation:** Aim for at least 150 minutes of moderate-intensity aerobic exercise per week, combined with strength training at least two days a week.

- **Adapt:** Modify exercise routines based on individual fitness levels and health conditions.

6. Bone-Loading Exercises:

- **Definition:** Bone-loading exercises involve activities that put stress on bones, promoting bone growth.

- **Examples:** Jumping jacks, hopping, and skipping can be effective bone-loading exercises.

7. Impact of Menopause and Aging:

- **Concern:** Bone density tends to decrease with age, especially in postmenopausal women.
- **Mitigation:** Regular weight-bearing exercises and strength training are particularly important for maintaining bone health as you age.

8. Nutrition and Exercise:

- **Calcium and Vitamin D:** Adequate intake of calcium and vitamin D is crucial for bone health. Ensure your diet supports your exercise routine.
- **Protein:** Protein is essential for bone formation and repair. Include sources of plant-based protein in your diet.

9. Rest and Recovery:

- **Importance:** Allow adequate time for rest and recovery between intense sessions.
- **Adaptation:** The body strengthens bones during rest periods, making recovery an integral part of the bone-building process.

10. Consultation with Healthcare Professionals:

- **Individual Considerations:** Consult with a healthcare professional or a fitness expert before starting a new exercise program, especially if you have pre-existing health conditions or concerns.

11. Maintaining a Healthy Lifestyle:

- **Avoiding Smoking and Excessive Alcohol:** Smoking and excessive alcohol consumption can negatively impact bone health. Maintaining a healthy lifestyle contributes to overall bone health.

Stress Reduction Techniques

Mindfulness and meditation can play a significant role in managing stress, which, in turn, may have positive effects on bone health. Let's explore the relationship between mindfulness, stress, and bone health:

Mindfulness and Meditation:

1. Definition:

- **Mindfulness:** A mental state of heightened awareness, focusing on the present moment without judgment.
- **Meditation:** A practice that involves training the mind to achieve a state of relaxed awareness.

2. Stress Reduction:

- Mindfulness and meditation techniques are proven methods for reducing stress and promoting relaxation.
- By fostering a calm and centered state of mind, these practices may help mitigate the negative effects of chronic stress.

3. Cortisol Regulation:

- Chronic stress can lead to elevated cortisol levels, which may contribute to bone loss.
- Mindfulness practices have been associated with improved cortisol regulation, potentially benefiting bone health.

4. Pain Management:

- Mindfulness meditation has been shown to be effective in managing chronic pain conditions.
- Chronic pain and discomfort can contribute to stress, and by alleviating pain, mindfulness may indirectly support bone health.

Impact of Stress on Bone Health:

1. Cortisol and Bone Resorption:

- Chronic stress can lead to increased cortisol production, which, in excess, is associated with higher bone resorption (breakdown).
- Elevated cortisol levels may interfere with the bone remodeling process and lead to decreased bone density.

2. Inflammation and Bone Health:

- Chronic stress may contribute to inflammation, and prolonged inflammation can negatively affect bone health.
- Inflammatory markers may influence the balance between bone formation and resorption.

3. Impact on Bone Mineral Density (BMD):

- Long-term exposure to stress may impact bone mineral density, making bones more susceptible to fractures.
- Stress-induced hormonal changes can affect the absorption of calcium and other minerals crucial for bone strength.

4. Behavioral Factors:

- Stress may contribute to unhealthy behaviors such as poor dietary choices, lack of physical activity, and disrupted sleep, all of which can affect bone health.

Integrating Mindfulness for Bone Health:

1. Regular Practice:

- Incorporate regular mindfulness or meditation sessions into your routine to manage stress levels.
- Apps, guided sessions, or classes can provide structured guidance.

2. Mindful Eating:

- Practice mindfulness during meals to promote healthier food choices and better digestion, providing nutrients essential for bone health.

3. Mind-Body Exercises:

- Engage in mind-body exercises like yoga or tai chi, which combine physical activity with mindfulness.

4. Quality Sleep:

- Mindfulness practices may improve sleep quality, positively impacting overall health, including bone health.

5. Stress Management Techniques:

- Learn and practice stress management techniques, such as deep breathing, progressive muscle relaxation, or guided imagery.

6. Professional Guidance:

- Consider seeking guidance from mindfulness instructors, therapists, or healthcare professionals to tailor practices to your specific needs.

CONCLUSION

Celebrating Your Journey to Healthier Bones:

Congratulations on embarking on the journey to maintain healthier bones through a plant-based lifestyle! Celebrate your accomplishments and commitment to overall well-being. As you reflect on your journey, here's a recap of key concepts and tips to continue your plant-based lifestyle:

Key Concepts Recap:

1. Understanding Osteoporosis:

- Gain knowledge about osteoporosis, its causes, and the importance of maintaining bone health through lifestyle choices.

2. Plant-Based Nutrition:

- Embrace a plant-based diet rich in calcium, vitamin D, magnesium, and other nutrients essential for bone health.
- Prioritize leafy greens, tofu, legumes, nuts, seeds, fortified plant milks, and whole grains.

3. Balanced Nutrient Intake:

- Pay attention to the balance of nutrients for optimal absorption, considering interactions between calcium, magnesium, vitamin D, and others.

4. Incorporating Calcium-Rich Foods:

- Include a variety of calcium-rich foods such as leafy greens, tofu, fortified plant milks, and nuts in your daily meals.

5. Vitamin D and Sunlight Exposure:

- Understand the importance of sunlight exposure for vitamin D synthesis and consider supplementation if needed.
- Include vitamin D-rich foods like mushrooms, fortified plant milks, and exposure to sunlight.

6. Balancing Nutrients for Optimal Absorption:

- Be mindful of nutrient interactions and balance your diet to maximize absorption.
- Consider consulting a healthcare professional or a dietitian for personalized advice.

7. Physical Activity and Bone Health:

- Incorporate weight-bearing exercises, strength training, and activities that promote balance and stability into your routine.
- Aim for a balanced and varied exercise regimen that suits your fitness level.

8. Mindfulness and Meditation:

- Recognize the impact of stress on bone health and incorporate mindfulness and meditation practices into your routine for stress reduction.
- Cultivate a mindful approach to eating and engage in activities that promote relaxation.

9. Celebrating Achievements:

- Acknowledge and celebrate your achievements, no matter how small.
- Regularly assess your progress and make adjustments to your lifestyle as needed.

Continuing Your Plant-Based Lifestyle:

1. Stay Informed:

- Stay updated on new developments in plant-based nutrition and bone health research.

2. Diversify Your Diet:

- Explore new plant-based recipes and ingredients to keep your meals exciting and nutritionally diverse.

3. Regular Check-ups:

- Schedule regular check-ups with healthcare professionals to monitor your bone health and overall well-being.

4. Adapt Your Exercise Routine:

- Adjust your exercise routine as needed, considering changes in fitness levels, preferences, and potential health conditions.

5. Mindful Living:

- Continue to cultivate mindfulness and stress-reduction practices in various aspects of your life.

6. Community Support:

- Join plant-based communities or support groups to share experiences, tips, and inspiration with like-minded individuals.

7. Set New Goals:

- Set new health and wellness goals to keep your journey dynamic and motivating.

Remember, the key to a sustainable and successful plant-based lifestyle is consistency and adaptability. Celebrate the positive changes you've made, and continue to prioritize your bone health and overall well-being. Your commitment to a plant-based lifestyle is an investment in your long-term health and vitality.

Appendix

Quick Reference Guide:

Nutrient Charts:

1. Calcium-Rich Foods:

- Kale: 1 cup cooked = 179 mg
- Tofu (firm, calcium-set): 1/2 cup = 861 mg
- Fortified Almond Milk: 1 cup = 300 mg
- Chia Seeds: 2 tablespoons = 179 mg
- Broccoli: 1 cup cooked = 62 mg

2. Vitamin D-Rich Foods:

- Fortified Orange Juice: 1 cup = 137 IU
- Portobello Mushrooms (exposed to sunlight): 1 cup sliced = 493 IU
- Fortified Plant Yogurt: 1 cup = 120 IU
- Sunflower Seeds: 1 ounce = 37 IU

3. Magnesium-Rich Foods:

- Almonds: 1 ounce = 76 mg
- Spinach: 1 cup cooked = 157 mg

- Pumpkin Seeds: 1 ounce = 150 mg
- Black Beans: 1 cup cooked = 120 mg
- Quinoa: 1 cup cooked = 118 mg

Sample Meal Plans:

Day 1:

Breakfast:

- Green Calcium Boost Smoothie
- **Ingredients:** Kale, banana, chia seeds, fortified almond milk

Lunch:

- Quinoa Salad with Chickpeas, Spinach, and Almonds
- **Dressing:** Olive oil, lemon juice, salt, and pepper

Dinner:

- Tofu Stir-Fry with Broccoli and Brown Rice
- **Sauce:** Soy sauce, ginger, garlic

Day 2:

Breakfast:

- Berry Bliss Calcium Smoothie
- **Ingredients:** Mixed berries, silken tofu, almond butter, fortified soy milk

Lunch:

- Lentil and Vegetable Soup
- **Ingredients:** Lentils, carrots, celery, tomatoes, spinach

Dinner:

- Baked Stuffed Bell Peppers with Quinoa and Black Beans
- **Toppings:** Avocado slices, salsa

Day 3:

Breakfast:

- Tropical Vitamin C Smoothie
- **Ingredients:** Pineapple, mango, kale, hemp seeds, coconut water

Lunch:

- Chickpea and Spinach Curry
- Serve with brown rice

Dinner:

- Grilled Portobello Mushrooms with Sunflower Seed Pesto

Side: Steamed broccoli

Note:

- Adjust portion sizes based on individual dietary needs and preferences.
- Incorporate snacks such as nuts, seeds, or fresh fruit as desired.
- Stay hydrated with water, herbal teas, or infused water throughout the day.